QUICK AND EASY FITNESS

A Guide to 10-Minute Daily Workouts for Seniors

Dr. Laurie Miles

<u>Other Books by The Author:</u>

•	Pilates for a Better 60+: A Guide to Safe and Effective Exercise for Seniors

•	Chair Yoga for Seniors Over 50: A Comprehensive Guide to Improving Health and Mobility for Active Aging

•	Stay Young at Heart: A Daily Workout Plan for Active Seniors + 14-Day Sample Workout Plan

INTRODUCTION

As we age, it becomes increasingly important to maintain a healthy and active lifestyle. Regular exercise not only helps keep our bodies strong and mobile, but it also has numerous mental and emotional benefits. Unfortunately, many seniors find it difficult to make time for regular workouts, or are intimidated by the thought of starting an exercise routine. But what if we told you that you could reap the benefits of exercise in just 10 minutes a day?

Quick and Easy Fitness is a comprehensive guide to daily workouts specifically designed for seniors. In this book, we'll show you how 10-minute daily workouts can improve your physical and mental health, and help prevent or manage age-related conditions such as arthritis, osteoporosis, and cardiovascular disease. We'll provide step-by-step instructions for a variety of workouts that can be completed in just 10 minutes, including warm-up exercises, strength-training exercises, cardiovascular exercises, and stretching and flexibility exercises.

Whether you're new to exercise or looking to add more activity to your daily routine, Quick and Easy Fitness makes it easy to get started. We'll provide tips for making exercise a daily habit, staying motivated, and overcoming obstacles. And we'll show you how to fit 10-minute workouts into your busy schedule, so you can experience the benefits of exercise without sacrificing your time and energy.

So, if you're ready to take control of your health and wellness, and start enjoying the benefits of daily exercise, Quick and Easy Fitness is the perfect guide for you!

Chapter 1
Introduction to Daily Workouts for Seniors

<u>Overview of the Importance of Daily Exercise for Seniors</u>

As seniors, it is essential to prioritize our physical and mental health. Regular exercise can play a crucial role in maintaining and improving both, but many seniors struggle to find the time and motivation to stick to a workout routine. The good news is that even just 10 minutes of daily exercise can have a profound impact on our well-being.

Physical activity has a plethora of benefits for seniors, including improved muscle strength and flexibility, better cardiovascular health, and reduced risk of age-related conditions like osteoporosis and arthritis. Additionally, regular exercise has been shown to improve mental health and cognitive function, boost mood and self-esteem, and help regulate sleep patterns.

The key to making exercise a regular part of our routine is to find activities that are manageable and enjoyable. The 10-minute daily workouts outlined in this book are designed to be simple, accessible, and effective, and can be done from the comfort of your own home. Whether you're new to exercise or simply looking to add more activity to your daily routine, these workouts can help you improve your physical and mental health in a way that fits into your busy schedule.

So, let's get started on a journey towards a healthier, happier, and more active lifestyle. With Quick and Easy Fitness, you'll see just how easy it can be to incorporate daily exercise into your routine and enjoy the many benefits that come with it.

Explanation of 10-Minute Daily Workouts

The idea behind 10-minute daily workouts is simple: you don't need to spend hours at the gym to see results. In fact, just a few minutes of daily exercise can have a significant impact on your physical and mental health. The workouts in this book are designed to be quick, easy, and accessible, so that seniors can fit them into their busy schedules without sacrificing time or energy.

So, what exactly are 10-minute daily workouts? They are short, targeted exercises that can be done in just 10 minutes a day, but are still effective at improving strength, flexibility, and overall fitness. These workouts are designed to be completed in sequence, with each exercise building upon the previous one. The workouts can be modified to accommodate different fitness levels, and can be done with minimal equipment or no equipment at all.

The benefits of 10-minute daily workouts are many. They are a great way to stay active, even when you're short on time. They can also help improve your overall health, including your cardiovascular health, strength, flexibility, and balance. Furthermore, 10-minute daily workouts are a great way to relieve stress, boost mood, and improve sleep quality.

So, whether you're new to exercise or simply looking to add more activity to your daily routine, 10-minute daily workouts are a great option. With Quick and Easy Fitness, you'll see just how easy it can be to incorporate daily exercise into your routine and enjoy the many benefits that come with it. So, let's get started!

Chapter 2
The Benefits of Daily Exercise for Seniors

<u>Physical Health Benefits</u>

Regular physical activity has numerous health benefits for seniors. Engaging in daily exercise can improve overall physical health, maintain independence, and prevent or manage chronic conditions. Some of the most significant physical health benefits of daily exercise for seniors include:

- **Improving Cardiovascular Health:**
Regular physical activity helps to increase heart health by lowering blood pressure and reducing the risk of heart disease. It also improves circulation, which can reduce the risk of stroke and other cardiovascular issues.

- **Strengthening Bones:**
As people age, bones can become more fragile and prone to osteoporosis. Regular exercise, especially weight-bearing exercises like walking and strength training, can help to maintain and even increase bone density.

- **Enhancing Balance and Coordination:**
Exercise can help to improve balance and coordination, reducing the risk of falls and related injuries. This is especially important for seniors, who are more likely to experience falls and related injuries.

- **Boosting Energy and Endurance:**
Regular exercise can help to increase energy levels, allowing seniors to participate in daily activities and maintain independence. Exercise can also help to improve endurance, allowing seniors to participate in longer and more strenuous physical activities.

- **Managing Chronic Conditions:**
Daily exercise can help to manage and even prevent chronic conditions like arthritis, diabetes, and cardiovascular disease. Regular exercise can help to reduce symptoms and manage related health issues.

- **Improving Mental Health:**
Regular exercise has been shown to have a positive impact on mental health, reducing stress and anxiety and improving mood. Engaging in daily exercise can help seniors to maintain a positive outlook and reduce feelings of isolation and loneliness.

- **Maintaining a Healthy Weight:**

Exercise can help to maintain a healthy weight, reducing the risk of obesity and related health issues. It also helps to improve metabolism, allowing seniors to more efficiently process food and maintain a healthy weight.

Mental Health Benefits of Daily Exercise for Seniors

Exercise has been proven time and time again to have a positive impact on mental health, and this is no different for seniors. Engaging in regular physical activity has been shown to reduce symptoms of depression and anxiety, improve overall mood, and boost self-esteem.

One of the key ways that exercise contributes to mental well-being is by increasing the release of endorphins in the brain. Endorphins are the body's natural feel-good chemicals that are released during physical activity and are known to reduce stress, anxiety, and depression. Seniors who engage in daily exercise can experience an improvement in their mood, sleep patterns, and overall mental health.

Another benefit of daily exercise is that it can help to keep the mind sharp and reduce the risk of cognitive decline as seniors age. Regular physical activity has been shown to improve memory, concentration, and cognitive function, which can be especially beneficial for seniors who may be experiencing age-related cognitive decline.

Furthermore, exercise can also provide a sense of structure and routine in seniors' lives, which can help to combat feelings of boredom, loneliness, and isolation. Joining an exercise group or taking part in community-based physical activities can also provide opportunities to socialize, meet new people, and stay connected with others, all of which are important factors in maintaining good mental health.

In conclusion, engaging in daily physical activity is not only good for the body, but it is also beneficial for the mind. Regular exercise has been shown to have a positive impact on mental health and well-being, including reducing symptoms of depression and anxiety, improving overall mood, and boosting self-esteem. Additionally, regular exercise can help to keep the mind sharp and reduce the risk of cognitive decline, provide a sense of structure and routine, and provide opportunities for socialization and staying connected with others.

Preventing and Managing Age-Related Conditions

Exercise is crucial for seniors as it plays a key role in preventing and managing age-related conditions. As we age, our bodies become more susceptible to various health problems such as arthritis, osteoporosis, and cardiovascular disease. By incorporating daily exercise into our lives, seniors can greatly reduce the risk of developing these conditions and improve their overall health.

Arthritis is a common age-related condition that affects millions of seniors. Regular physical activity, such as daily workouts, can help ease the pain associated with arthritis by improving joint flexibility and reducing inflammation.

Osteoporosis is a condition that weakens the bones and increases the risk of fractures. Weight-bearing exercises, such as those included in 10-minute daily workouts, can help to increase bone density and reduce the risk of osteoporosis.

Cardiovascular disease is another age-related condition that can be prevented and managed through daily exercise. Physical activity helps to lower blood pressure, improve cholesterol levels, and reduce the risk of heart disease. By incorporating 10-minute daily workouts into their routine, seniors can improve their cardiovascular health and reduce the risk of heart disease.

In addition to preventing and managing age-related conditions, daily exercise can also help to improve overall health and well-being. By taking just 10 minutes a day to engage in physical activity, seniors can enjoy numerous benefits and lead a healthier, more fulfilling life.

Chapter 3
Getting Started with 10-Minute Daily Workouts

<u>Equipment Needed</u>

Exercise equipment can range from minimal to extensive, but it is important to note that for 10-minute daily workouts, little to no equipment is necessary. For seniors, the most important piece of equipment is a sturdy pair of shoes to prevent falls and provide adequate support for their feet and ankles. Additionally, seniors may choose to invest in a simple exercise mat for added comfort and cushioning.

For strength training exercises, seniors can use light weights, resistance bands, or even household items such as water bottles or canned goods. Cardiovascular exercises can be performed without any equipment, such as walking or jumping jacks. However, if seniors have access to a stationary bike or treadmill, these can also be used for a more low-impact cardiovascular workout.

It is important for seniors to remember that exercise equipment is not a requirement for a successful workout. Instead, the focus should be on proper form and technique, which can be achieved with or without equipment. If seniors choose to invest in equipment, they should consider their budget, storage space, and any physical limitations they may have.

Overall, the key to a successful 10-minute daily workout is consistency, not the amount or type of equipment used. By committing to daily exercise, seniors can reap the numerous physical and mental health benefits, regardless of the equipment they have available.

Starting Slowly and Progressing Gradually

Starting slowly and progressing gradually is an important aspect of getting started with 10-minute daily workouts for seniors. This approach allows you to gradually build up your strength and endurance over time, reducing the risk of injury and helping you to achieve your fitness goals in a safe and sustainable way.

When you first start exercising, it's important to start with low-impact activities that are easy on your joints, such as walking, cycling, or swimming. You can gradually increase the intensity and duration of these activities as your fitness improves. For example, you might start with 10 minutes of walking each day, and gradually increase this to 20 or 30 minutes over the course of several weeks.

In addition to increasing the duration of your workouts, you should also aim to gradually increase the intensity. This can be done by adding weights, using resistance bands, or increasing the incline on a treadmill or stationary bike. As you get stronger, you can add more challenging exercises, such as lunges, squats, and push-ups, to your routine.

It's also important to listen to your body and not push yourself too hard, too fast. If you experience pain, discomfort, or fatigue, it's a sign that you need to take a break or slow down. Always consult with your doctor before starting a new exercise program, especially if you have any pre-existing medical conditions.

Starting slowly and progressing gradually is a smart and effective way to get started with 10-minute daily workouts for seniors. By following this approach, you'll be able to gradually build up your strength and endurance, and achieve your fitness goals in a safe and sustainable way.

Safety Tips for Seniors

Exercising is a great way to maintain good health and prevent injury, but as a senior, it's especially important to follow certain safety guidelines. Here are a few tips to keep in mind when starting your 10-minute daily workouts:

- **Consult with a doctor:**

Before starting any exercise program, it's always a good idea to consult with a doctor to make sure that you're in good health and able to exercise safely. Your doctor can also provide specific recommendations based on your individual health needs.

- **Warm up before each workout:**

Before beginning any physical activity, it's important to warm up your muscles. This helps to prepare your body for exercise and reduce the risk of injury. You can start with a gentle warm-up such as marching in place, arm circles or leg swings.

- **Use proper technique:**

When performing exercises, be sure to use proper technique to reduce the risk of injury. This includes using the correct form and alignment, moving slowly and smoothly, and avoiding any sudden, jerky movements.

- **Listen to your body:**

Pay attention to how your body feels during and after each workout. If you experience pain or discomfort, stop the exercise and rest. It's also important to pace yourself and not overdo it, especially in the beginning.

- **Wear the right footwear:**

Proper footwear can help prevent injury and ensure that you get the most out of your workout. Look for shoes with good support, cushioning and stability.

- **Stay hydrated:**

Staying hydrated is important during exercise, especially as a senior. Be sure to drink plenty of water before, during and after your workout to avoid dehydration.

By following these safety tips, you can exercise safely and enjoy the many benefits that come from staying active. With a little preparation and a commitment to taking care of your body, you can stay fit and healthy for years to come!

Chapter 4
10-Minute Daily Workouts

Gentle Warm-Up Exercises

Warming up before starting any form of physical activity is important, and especially so for seniors. A warm-up can help to prepare the body for exercise, reduce the risk of injury, and improve flexibility and range of motion. A gentle warm-up is also a great way to start your 10-minute daily workout.

Some effective warm-up exercises for seniors include:

- **Marching or walking in place:**
This is a great way to get the blood flowing and to prepare the muscles for more intense activities. You can start by marching in place for 2-3 minutes, and then gradually increase the intensity.

- **Shoulder rolls:**
Stand with your feet shoulder-width apart and your arms at your sides. Roll your shoulders backwards

and then forwards, repeating the motion for 2-3 minutes.

- **Neck rolls:**

Stand or sit with your arms relaxed at your sides. Gently roll your head from side to side, holding each position for a few seconds. Repeat the motion for 2-3 minutes.

- **Arm swings:**

Stand with your feet shoulder-width apart and your arms hanging loosely at your sides. Swing your arms backwards and then forwards, repeating the motion for 2-3 minutes.

- **Ankle circles:**

Stand with your feet shoulder-width apart and your arms relaxed at your sides. Gently rotate your ankles in a clockwise direction, then in an anti-clockwise direction. Repeat the motion for 2-3 minutes.

It's important to remember that warm-up exercises should be done at a low intensity, and should never cause pain or discomfort. You can also modify the exercises to suit your level of fitness and comfort. The main goal of the warm-up is to prepare the body for exercise and to reduce the risk of injury.

Strength-Training Exercises

Strength-training exercises are essential for seniors as they help to build and maintain muscle mass, improve balance, and prevent falls. These exercises can be done using light weights, resistance bands, or even your own body weight. The key is to start slowly and progress gradually, using proper form to avoid injury.

Some of the most effective strength-training exercises for seniors include:

- **Squats:**
Stand with your feet shoulder-width apart and your arms extended straight in front of you. Slowly lower your body as if you were sitting back into a chair, then push back up to the starting position.

- **Push-Ups:**
Get into a plank position, with your hands placed slightly wider than shoulder-width apart. Lower your body until your chest nearly touches the ground, then push back up to the starting position.

- **Bicep Curls:**

Hold a light weight in each hand and stand with your feet shoulder-width apart. Keep your elbows close to your sides as you lift the weights towards your shoulders, then slowly lower back down.

- **Triceps Dips:**

Sit on the edge of a chair or bench, with your hands placed beside you. Slide your bottom off the edge and lower your body until your arms form a 90-degree angle, then push back up to the starting position.

- **Leg Raises:**

Lie on your back with your legs extended straight up towards the ceiling. Slowly lower one leg towards the ground, then raise it back up to the starting position. Repeat with the other leg.

Remember, the goal of strength-training exercises is to challenge your muscles, not to exhaust them. It's important to start with light weights and work your way up as you build strength. Always listen to your body and never push yourself to the point of pain.

Incorporating strength-training exercises into your 10-minute daily workout routine will help to improve your overall physical health and prevent age-related conditions like osteoporosis, arthritis, and sarcopenia (the loss of muscle mass and strength that occurs as we age).

Cardiovascular Exercises

Cardiovascular exercises, also known as aerobic exercises, are an important component of a well-rounded fitness routine, and can be easily incorporated into a 10-minute daily workout. These exercises raise the heart rate and improve the function of the cardiovascular system, which helps to maintain a healthy heart, lungs, and blood vessels.

For seniors, engaging in cardiovascular exercises can provide a range of health benefits, including:

- Improved heart and lung function
- Reduced risk of heart disease, stroke, and other chronic conditions
- Better blood flow, which helps to prevent clogged arteries and reduces the risk of developing blood clots
- Increased energy levels, making it easier to perform daily activities
- Improved endurance, which can help to reduce fatigue and improve overall quality of life.

There are many different types of cardiovascular exercises that can be performed within the constraints of a 10-minute workout. Some popular options include:

- **Walking:**

A simple, low-impact exercise that is easy on the joints and can be performed almost anywhere.

- **Cycling**:

A fun, low-impact exercise that can be performed indoors or outdoors, depending on the weather and personal preferences.

- **Dancing:**

A fun way to incorporate movement into a daily workout, dancing is also a great way to improve coordination, balance, and overall cardiovascular health.

- **Chair aerobics:**

A low-impact exercise that can be performed from a seated position, making it an ideal choice for seniors with mobility issues.

- **Aqua aerobics:**

A fun, low-impact exercise performed in a swimming pool, perfect for those who enjoy being in the water.

Regardless of the specific exercise chosen, it's important to start slowly and gradually increase the intensity as physical condition improves. It's also a good idea to talk to a doctor before starting a new exercise program, especially if there are any underlying health conditions. With regular exercise and a healthy diet, seniors can enjoy improved physical and mental health, and maintain an active and fulfilling lifestyle well into their golden years.

Stretching and Flexibility Exercises

Stretching and flexibility exercises are important components of any workout routine, especially for seniors. As we age, our muscles and joints become less flexible and more prone to injury. Incorporating stretching and flexibility exercises into your 10-minute daily workout can help improve your range of motion, prevent injury, and keep your muscles and joints in good condition.

There are many types of stretching and flexibility exercises that can be done in a short amount of time, including static stretching, dynamic stretching, and foam rolling.

Static stretching involves holding a stretch for a specific amount of time, usually 20-30 seconds. This type of stretching is great for increasing flexibility and reducing muscle tension. Dynamic stretching, on the other hand, involves moving through a range of motion in a controlled manner, which helps prepare your muscles for activity. Foam rolling is a form of self-massage that can be used to relieve muscle tightness and improve flexibility.

When incorporating stretching and flexibility exercises into your 10-minute daily workout, it's important to warm up first. A gentle warm-up such as a light walk or some easy stretches can prepare your body for the stretching exercises.

Some great stretching and flexibility exercises for seniors include:

- Hamstring stretches
- Quad stretches
- Hip flexor stretches
- Shoulder stretches
- Lower back stretches
- Calf stretches

- Yoga poses like the downward dog, cat-cow, and warrior

There are various stretching exercises that can be done in just a few minutes each day, including:

- **Hamstring stretch:**
Sit on the floor with both legs extended in front of you, reach forward and try to touch your toes. Hold for 10-15 seconds and release.

- **Upper back stretch:**
Stand with your feet hip-width apart and clasp your hands behind your back, lift your arms and hold for 10-15 seconds.

- **Arm and shoulder stretch:**
Stand with your feet hip-width apart, reach one arm across your chest and hold it with the opposite hand. Hold for 10-15 seconds, release and repeat on the other side.

- **Calf stretch:**
Stand facing a wall with both hands on it and one foot behind the other. Keep the back leg straight and the front knee bent, hold for 10-15 seconds, release and repeat on the other side.

- **Quad Stretches:**

Quad stretches help to loosen the muscles located in the front of the thigh. To perform a quad stretch, stand with your feet hip-width apart and hold onto a wall or chair for balance. Bend your knee and bring your heel towards your buttocks, then grab your ankle with your hand. Hold the stretch for 20 to 30 seconds, then release and repeat on the other leg.

- **Hip Flexor Stretches:**

The hip flexors are a group of muscles located at the front of the hip and are often tight due to sitting for extended periods of time. To perform a hip flexor stretch, kneel on the ground with one knee bent and the other leg extended behind you. Lean forward, keeping your back straight, until you feel a stretch in the front of your hip. Hold the stretch for 20 to 30 seconds, then repeat on the other side.

- **Yoga Poses:**

Yoga poses, such as the downward-facing dog, cat and cow, and the warrior series, can help to increase flexibility and mobility in the muscles of the legs, hips, and lower back. These poses should be performed slowly and with proper form to prevent injury. Before attempting any new yoga poses, it is important to consult with a physician or licensed yoga instructor to determine if they are appropriate for your individual needs.

It's important to warm up before stretching to prevent injury, and to hold each stretch for at least 10-15 seconds for maximum benefit. Remember to listen to your body, and never push yourself beyond your limits.

Remember, consistency is key. Incorporating stretching and flexibility exercises into your 10-minute daily workout can help you maintain good mobility, prevent injury, and feel great.

Tips for Making the Most of Each Workout

Making the most of your 10-minute daily workout is key to getting the most benefits from your exercise routine. Here are a few tips to help you get the most out of each workout:

- **Set a goal:**

Before starting your workout, set a goal for what you hope to achieve. This could be anything from increasing your strength to improving your flexibility. Having a goal will give you something to work towards and will help you stay motivated.

- **Warm up:**

Make sure to start each workout with a gentle warm-up. This will help you to prepare your body for exercise, reduce the risk of injury, and improve your performance.

- **Focus on form:**

Pay close attention to your form when performing each exercise. Poor form can lead to injury, and can also mean that you are not getting the full benefit of each exercise.

- **Mix it up:**

To keep your workouts interesting and challenging, try to mix things up by doing a variety of exercises. This will help you to work different muscle groups and keep you engaged and motivated.

- **Track your progress:**

Keeping track of your progress is important, as it can help you to see how far you've come and motivate you to keep going. Write down the exercises you do, how many repetitions you perform, and how much weight you use. You can also track other aspects of your fitness, such as your body measurements, strength, and flexibility.

- **Stay consistent:**

Consistency is key when it comes to achieving your fitness goals. Make sure to exercise every day, and try to stick to your routine as much as possible.

By following these tips, you can maximize the benefits of your 10-minute daily workouts and achieve your fitness goals

Chapter 5
Making Exercise a Habit

Creating a Daily Routine

Exercise is a crucial part of maintaining physical and mental health, especially as we age. However, turning exercise into a habit can be a challenge, especially when other responsibilities, such as work and caring for loved ones, consume our time and energy. Fortunately, there are steps you can take to make exercise a regular part of your routine.

Here are some tips for creating a daily exercise routine:

- **Make it a priority:**
Exercise should be one of your top priorities, along with eating well and getting enough sleep. Schedule your workouts for the same time each day, just like you would any other important appointment.

- **Start small:**
If you are new to exercise, or haven't been active for a while, start with 10-minute workouts and gradually increase the length and intensity of your sessions.

- **Choose activities you enjoy:**

The key to sticking with a workout routine is finding activities you enjoy. If you don't like running, try swimming, cycling, or yoga. If you don't enjoy the gym, try working out at home or in a park.

- **Mix it up:**

Doing the same exercises every day can quickly become monotonous. Mix up your routine by trying new exercises, joining a group fitness class, or working out with a partner.

- **Track your progress:**

Keeping track of your progress can help you stay motivated. Write down your workouts, the exercises you do, and how you feel after each session. Reviewing your progress regularly can help you see how far you have come and how much further you can go.

- **Be consistent:**

Consistency is key when it comes to creating a daily exercise routine. Don't get discouraged if you miss a day or two, just get back on track as soon as you can.

Remember, the goal is to make exercise a habit, not a chore. With these tips, you can create a daily routine that is both effective and enjoyable.

Staying Motivated

Staying motivated to exercise on a daily basis can be a challenge, especially for seniors who may have less energy or be dealing with health issues. However, there are several strategies that can help keep seniors motivated and on track with their fitness goals.

One key to staying motivated is setting realistic, achievable goals. Rather than focusing on losing a large amount of weight or gaining significant muscle, seniors can start by setting goals to improve their overall health, such as increasing energy levels or reducing joint pain. This can help them see progress and feel a sense of accomplishment along the way.

Another effective strategy is to find an exercise buddy. Having someone to exercise with can provide accountability, encouragement, and support. Seniors can work out with a friend, family member, or even a professional trainer. Exercising with others can also be more fun and help make the experience more enjoyable.

Incorporating variety into one's exercise routine can also help keep seniors motivated. This can mean trying new exercises or activities, changing up the time of day for workouts, or setting different goals for each workout. Mixing things up can help prevent boredom and keep seniors engaged in their fitness journey.

Seniors can also stay motivated by tracking their progress. This can be done by keeping a journal or using a fitness app to record progress and set new goals. Seeing the progress, they've made can be a great source of motivation and encouragement.

Finally, it's important for seniors to have a positive attitude and stay focused on the long-term benefits of exercise. Regular physical activity can help improve overall health and well-being, reduce the risk of chronic disease, and improve quality of life. By keeping this in mind, seniors can stay motivated to continue their fitness journey and reap the numerous benefits of daily exercise.

Overcoming Obstacles

Exercising regularly can bring numerous benefits to seniors, but the journey can be challenging and require overcoming various obstacles. Some seniors may face physical limitations that make exercise difficult, while others may struggle with a lack of motivation or difficulty making time for daily workouts. Here are some strategies for overcoming these obstacles:

- **Physical limitations:**

If you have physical limitations that make exercise challenging, it's important to consult a doctor and/or physical therapist. They can help you identify safe and effective exercises that are suitable for your needs, as well as provide modifications and adaptations. If you have mobility issues, you may want to consider exercises that can be performed while seated, such as chair yoga, or exercises that focus on upper body strength, such as weightlifting.

- **Lack of motivation:**

Staying motivated can be difficult, especially if you're not seeing immediate results. To keep yourself motivated, set achievable goals and track your progress. Surround yourself with supportive friends and family members who encourage you and celebrate your successes. You can also join a fitness class, hire a personal trainer, or find a workout partner who can help you stay on track.

- **Time constraints:**

Many seniors have busy schedules, making it difficult to carve out time for daily workouts. To overcome this obstacle, try to schedule your workouts at the same time each day. This can help you build a routine and make it easier to stick to your exercise regimen. You can also consider incorporating physical activity into your daily routine, such as taking a walk during your lunch break, using the stairs instead of the elevator, or doing light stretching during commercial breaks while watching TV.

- **Fear of injury or pain:**

Some seniors may be worried about the risk of injury or experience pain during exercise. To overcome this obstacle, it's important to start slowly and progress gradually, as well as engage in low-impact exercises that are safe and easy on the joints. You may also want to consider using props, such as foam rollers, to help reduce pain or discomfort.

Remember, overcoming obstacles and sticking to a regular exercise routine can bring numerous benefits, including improved physical and mental health, and the prevention and management of age-related conditions. With a little perseverance and a positive attitude, you can make exercise a daily habit that provides you with a lifetime of health and wellness benefits.

Fitting Exercise into a Busy Schedule

For many seniors, the biggest challenge to starting a daily exercise routine is finding the time. With so many other demands on their time and energy, it can be difficult to prioritize exercise. However, there are several strategies you can use to fit exercise into even the busiest of schedules.

First, consider breaking up your exercise into smaller chunks. Instead of trying to find a block of 30-60 minutes for a workout, you can split it into two 15-minute sessions or even three 10-minute sessions. This makes it easier to find the time and eliminates the pressure to make a large time commitment.

Another strategy is to look for opportunities to incorporate physical activity into your daily routine. For example, you can take the stairs instead of the elevator, park further away from the entrance to a store, or take a walk after dinner. These small changes can add up and help you get the physical activity you need.

It's also important to be flexible and adaptable. If you're not able to exercise at your usual time one day, don't be discouraged. Instead, try to find another time that works for you or adjust your routine accordingly.

In addition, it can be helpful to enlist the support of friends and family. Exercising with a friend can help make the time fly by and provide motivation to stick to your routine.

Ultimately, fitting exercise into a busy schedule is about finding what works for you and making it a priority. Whether you choose to work out first thing in the morning, during your lunch break, or after dinner, the important thing is to make it a regular part of your routine. With some planning and flexibility, you can find a way to fit exercise into your busy schedule and enjoy the numerous benefits that come with it.

CONCLUSION

In conclusion, incorporating daily exercise into your routine as a senior can have numerous physical and mental health benefits, as well as prevent and manage age-related conditions. 10-minute daily workouts are a great starting point and can be done with minimal equipment while following safety guidelines. The workouts should consist of warm-up, strength training, cardiovascular, and stretching exercises. To make exercise a habit, it's important to create a daily routine, stay motivated, overcome obstacles, and fit it into your busy schedule. Regular exercise can improve overall well-being and lead to a happier and healthier life.